Herbs That Cure

Eye Problems

Time-Tested Herbal Remedies

No Side-effects

by

Prayank

Contents

13. Lime for eye disease, watery in eyes

14. Liquorice for eye aching, to remove yellowness

15. Onion for eyesight weakness

16. Papaya for eye disease

17. Rose for burning sensation in eyes

18. Saunf for eye inflammation, irritation, eye strain due to excessive reading or TV watching, strengthen eye muscles

19. Sesame for burning sensation in eyes

20. Sweet Basil for boil on eyelids

21. Tamarind for eye diseases, redness, swelling in eyes

22. Turmeric for eye diseases, ophthalmia

23. Vasaka for eye diseases

24. Vibhitaki for imparting brightness in eyes

Some Important Guidelines

Introduction

Eye problems can be a serious threat to vision if not treated appropriately and in a timely fashion. The most obvious presentation of ocular (eye) trouble is redness and pain of the affected eyes. Health of the eyes and related structures, as well as vision must be taken care of at all times.

In the book, you will find brief details of herbs that can be used for eye care. It also gives you an option to choose the herb that is easily available in your locality. Herb names may be different in different places, hence you should rely on botanical names to find how it is known in a particular place/location.

Though there are people who treat ailments inexpensively with herbal remedies, most consider it as the last minute miracle worker once all other avenues of treatments have been exhausted.

Such an approach discounts the sophisticated and elaborately documented information dealing with specific medicinal applications of herbs for specific complaints. The methods of herbal remedies are designed for optimum beneficial use and tested innumerable times in actual practice.

While every effort has been made to verify the authenticity of information contained in this book, it is not intended as a substitute for medicinal consultation with a physician. The publisher and the author are in no way liable for the use of information contained in the book.

1. <u>Aloe</u>

(Aloe vera)

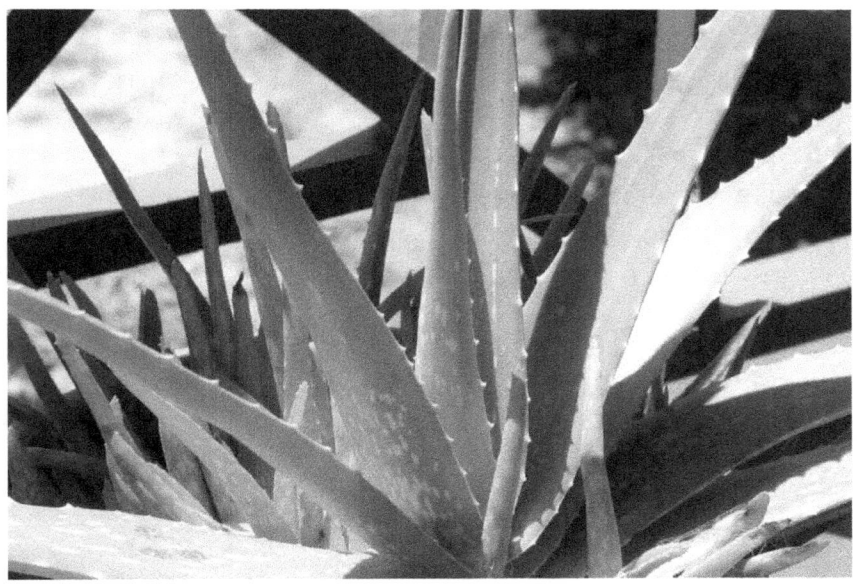

General

Aloe is a species of succulent plant that bears thorny lance-like leaves but is a favorite herb in beauty products. The fresh juice from leaves is yellowish in colour but acquires a brownish black colour on drying. The pulp is quite bitter to taste, and emits a somewhat offensive smell. It contains the active principle aloins.

Profile

Botanical Name : Aloe vera

Other Species : Aloe barbadenesis

Family : Liliaceae

Appearance : The fibrous root produces a rosette of succulent, lance-like leaves, whitish green on both sides with spines on the margins. Flowers - orange or yellow to purplish, in racemes. Fruit - a triangular capsule, ellipsoid-oblong.

Medicinal Parts : The gel-like pulp obtained on peeling the leaves and its dried form (powder); leaves.

Distribution : Widely cultivated throughout the world.

Ailments and Cure

Irritation in the eyes – Dissolve ½ tsp aloe and 1 tsp boric acid in 1 cup water. Use the solution as an eyewash. (Caution: Take all hygiene measures to avoid infection.)

Redness of eyes – Scoop out the pulp and bandage over the eyelids before going to bed. Repeat for 3 days.

2. Amla

(Phyllanthus emblica)

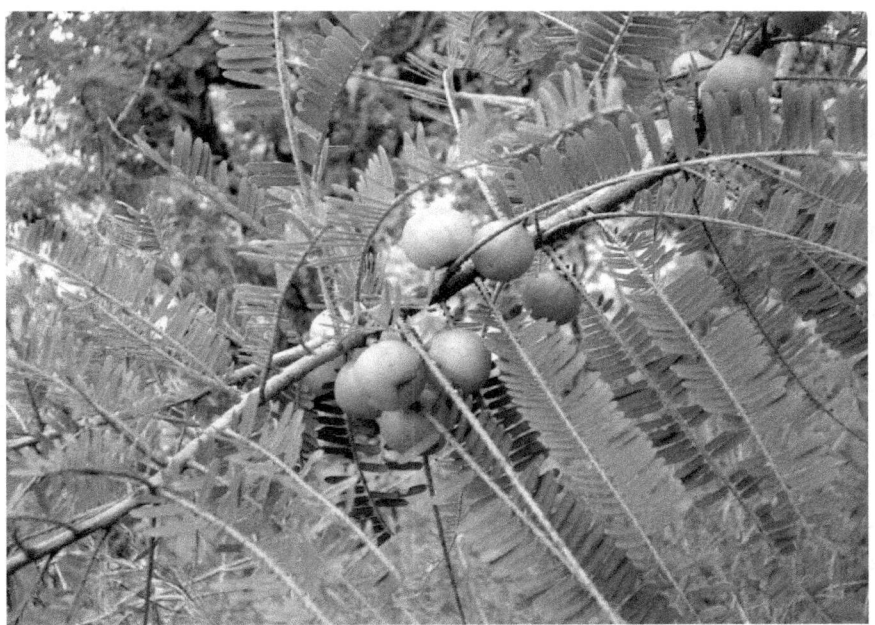

General

It is said that one can survive by consuming the fruit juice of amla only. It is the richest source of vitamin C, providing 3000mg of vitamin C per 100g of dried amla, which is heat stable.

There are two varieties of amla : the wild one with small fruits, and the cultivated ones with bigger fruits. Both are known to possess medicinal value.

Profile

Botanical Name : Phyllanthus emblica

Other Species : Emblica officinalis

Family : Euphorbiaceae

Appearance : A medium tree with smooth greenish-gray exfoliating bark. Leaves – feathery. Fruits – globose pale green, 1-5 cm in diameter, fleshy, sour in taste, 6-lobed.

Medicinal Parts : Fruits, leaves, flowers, seeds, root and bark.

Distribution : Native to India. It is present throughout tropical and sub-tropical regions up to 1500 m.

Ailments and Cure

Eye problems, night blindness - Crush fresh amla fruit along with a little water and express about 2 teacups juice. Add to this equal quantity of cow's milk and juice of trailing eclipta (marsh daisy). Add 8 teacups coconut water and 6 teacups sesame oil. Mix in 3 tsp each fine powder of following separately:Liquorice, wild turmeric, nutmeg, mace, chebulic myrobalan, belleric myrobalan, dried ginger and black pepper.

Now mix all the ingredients together in a vessel and heat over low flame. When the mixture reduces in volume and looses all traces of moisture, leaving behind a thick oil, remove from the fire. Allow it to cool. Bottle it.

Use 2-3 tsp of this oil to apply on scalp. Massage with fingers for 10 minutes. Wash it off with warm water.

3. <u>Bael</u>

<u>*(Aegle marmelos)*</u>

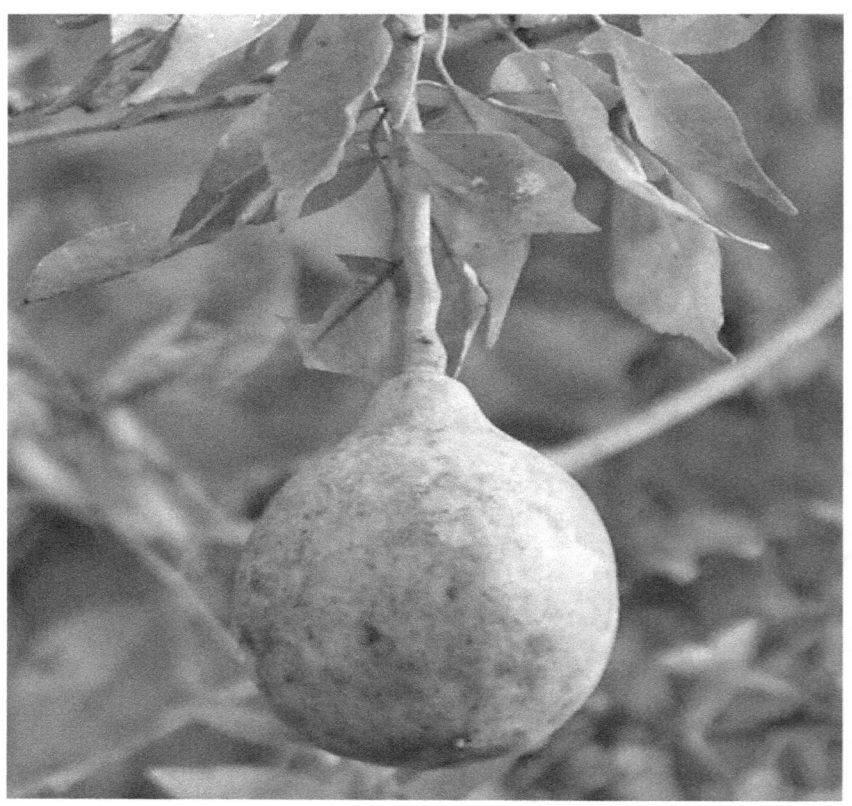

General

Bilva or bael tree (also known as Bengal quince, stone apple or wood apple) is native to India. The tree is considered to be sacred by Hindus. Its fruits are used in traditional medicine and as a food throughout its range.

Profile

Botanical Name : Aegle marmelos

Other Species : Crataeva marmelos

Family : Rutaceae

Appearance : Thorny tree with edible ripe fruits. Leaves are tri-foliate. Flowers – greenish-white, sweet-smelling, and in small bunches. Fruit – large and round with greenish-gray woody shell. Pulp inside is orange in color with many seeds covered with fibrous hairs, aromatic.

Medicinal Parts : Root, bark, leaves, flowers, and fruit.

Distribution : Native to India. It is present throughout Southeast Asia as a naturalized species.

Ailments and Cure

Eye disease, redness in eyes – Pluck a handful of tender leaf buds and roast in a mud pot. Tie them in a muslin cloth and apply on eyelids, when bearably warm.

Burning sensation in eyes – Take 3 tbsp each of fruit pulp of bael, babchi (Psoralea coryllifolia) and fenugreek. Add 1 teacup milk and grind into a fine paste. Add this to 2 teacups sesame oil and boil thoroughly. Cool, filter and store in a bottle. Apply this oil on the head and massage well before a shower.

4. <u>Banana</u>

(Musa paradisiaca)

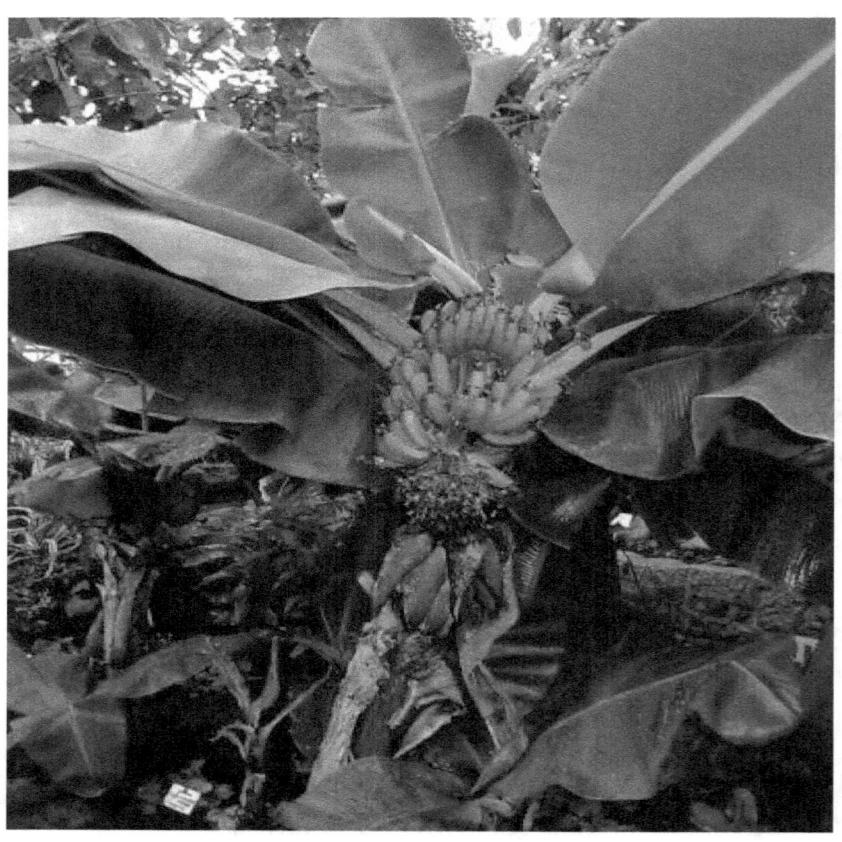

General

The term "banana" is used as the common name for the plants which produce the fruit, and the fruit itself. Fruits (unripe or ripe) and the edible rootstock have several curative properties.

Profile

Botanical Name : Musa paradisiaca, Musa sapientuum

Family : Musaceau

Appearance : A tall herb with aerial pseudo stem, dying after flowering. Leaves – large, oblong, narrowed to base. Flowers – in spikes, drooping with conspicuous bracts, dull brown. Fruits – in several clusters, generally golden yellow on ripening.

Medicinal Parts : Root, stem, sheath, leaves, flower, fruits.

Distribution : Native to tropical South and Southeast Asia, they are now grown in at least 107 countries, primarily for their fruit, and to a lesser extent to make fiber, banana wine and as ornamental plants.

Ailments and Cure

Burning sensation in eyes – Mash 1 ripe banana along with a little curd and water. Take twice a day.

5. <u>Banyan</u>

(Ficus benghalensis)

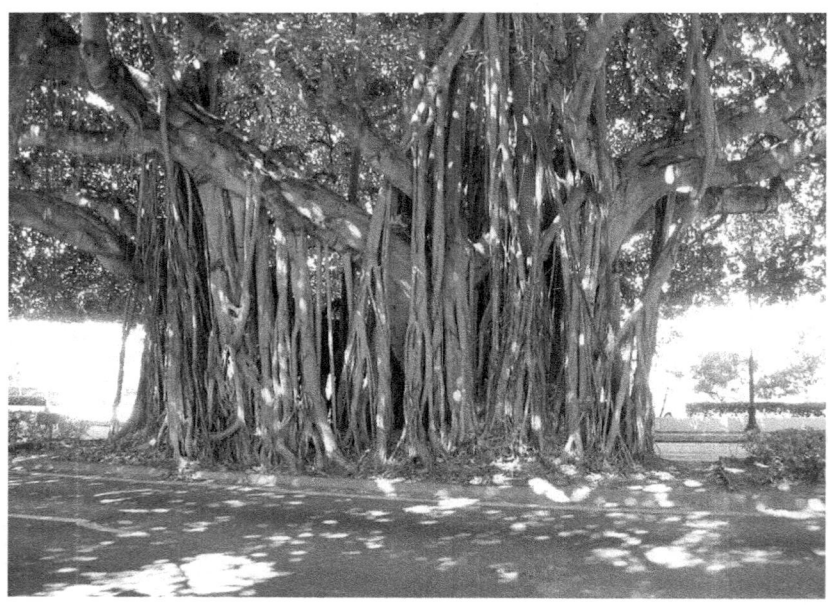

General

"Banyan" often refers specifically to the Indian banyan or
Ficus benghalensis. The seeds of banyans are dispersed by
fruit-eating birds. The seeds germinate and send down roots
towards the ground, and may envelop part of the host tree or
building structure with their roots.

Older banyan trees are characterized by their aerial prop roots that grow into thick woody trunks which, with age, can become indistinguishable from the main trunk. Old trees can spread out laterally using these prop roots to cover a wide area.

Profile

Botanical Name : Ficus benghalensis

Other Species : Urostig benghalense

Family : Moraceae

Appearance : A large tree with aerial roots. Leaves - large, leathery and oval, deep green above and pale green below. Young leaves have an attractive reddish tinge.

Medicinal Parts : .It is a milk-exuding tree. Several parts of this tree - stem bark, root bark, aerial roots, leaves, vegetative buds, sap (milk exudate), flowers, fruits find their use in herbal medicine.

Distribution : All over India - from sea level up to an altitude of 1000 m.

Ailments and Cure

Conjunctivitis, Gritty feeling in eyes, ophthalmia – Grind together one clove and sticky juice of banyan tree into a very fine paste. Wrap in a clean muslin. Squeeze the drops into eyes. (Note: 1. Take necessary hygiene precautions to prevent infection. 2. This may cause irritation in eyes.)

6. <u>Black Cumin</u>

(Nigella sativa)

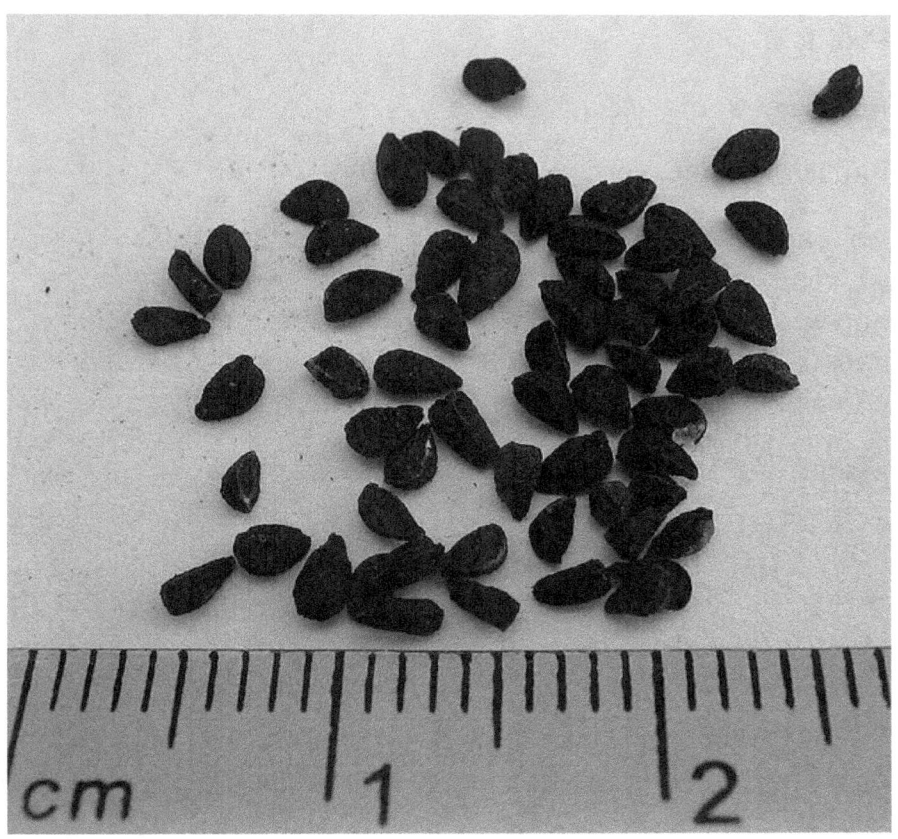

General

Black cumin is dried seed-like fruit of a small herb originally from Mediterranean region. It is stimulant, carminative and diuretic.

Profile

Botanical Name : Nigella sativa

Family : Ranunculaceae

Appearance : An annual flowering plant up to 20–30 cm tall, with finely divided, linear leaves. Flowers delicate, pale blue and white, with five to ten petals. Fruit is a large and inflated capsule composed of three to seven united follicles, each containing numerous seeds. Seeds black, trigonous.

Medicinal Parts : Seeds

Distribution: Native to south and southwest Asia.

Ailments and Cure

Yellow pigmentation in eyes due to jaundice – Grind ¼ tsp black cumin seeds in breast milk and introduce a pinch into nostrils.

7. <u>Cardamom</u>

(Elettaria cardamomum)

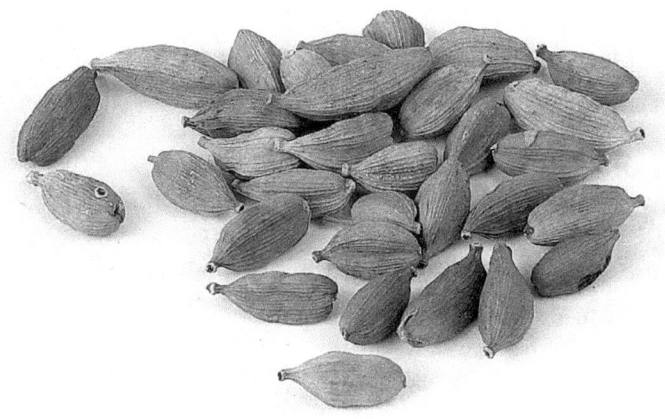

General

Cardamom awakens the spleen, stimulates the heart and imparts clarity and peace of mind. It possesses digestive, antispasmodic and carminative (helps dispel flatus) properties. It helps to stop belching, vomiting or acid regurgitation. It relieves spasms, induces perspiration and restores circulation.

When added to milk it neutralizes its mucus forming properties. It also detoxifies the caffeine in coffee.

Profile

Botanical Name : Elettaria Cardamomum

Family : Zingiberaceae

Appearance : A herb with fleshy branched rhizome. Leaves very large, narrow. Flowering stock arises from the base of the stem.

Medicinal Parts : Seeds

Distribution: Native to southeastern Asia from India south to SriLanka and east to Malaysia and western Indonesia, where it grows in tropical rainforests.

Ailments and Cure

Eyesight weakness – Mix seeds of cardamom along with 1 tbsp honey. Eat every day.

8. <u>Castor</u>

(Ricinus communis)

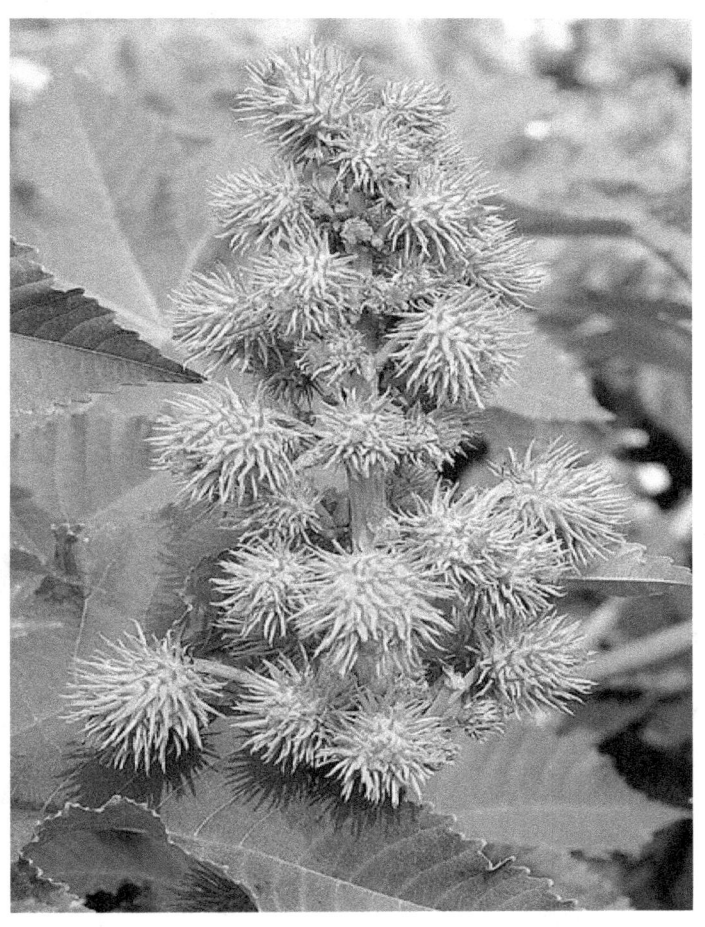

General

Castor seed is the source of castor oil, which has a wide variety of uses. The seeds contain between 40% and 60% oil that is rich in triglycerides, mainly ricinolein. The seed contains ricin, a toxin, which is also present in lower concentrations throughout the plant.

Medicinally, castor oil is a strong purgative.

Profile

Botanical Name : Ricinus communis

Other Species : white seeded castor, pale seeded castor

Family : Euphorbiaceae

Appearance : A tree like shrub, herbaceous, 3 to 10 feet tall. Leaves - palm like. Fruit - spiny capsule. Seeds - glossy.

Medicinal Parts : Leaves, seeds, roots, oil from seeds

Distribution: Castor is indigenous to the southeastern Mediterranean Basin, Eastern Africa, and India, but is widespread throughout tropical regions.

Ailments and Cure

Eye diseases - Instil 1 or 2 drops of infusion of the leaves in the eye. (Caution :Take all precautions to prevent infection.)

Burning sensation, pain in eyes – Apply castor oil over eyelashes before going to sleep.

Redness in eyes due to pollution or due to medication – Mix a little breast milk in castor oil and apply on the eyes at bedtime.

9. Durva

(Cynodon dactylon)

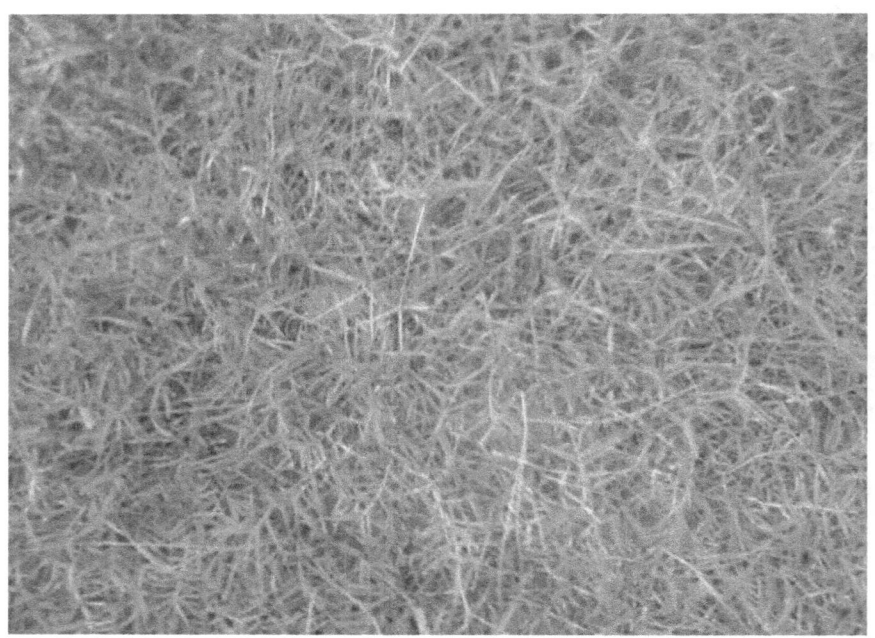

General

Full of chlorophyll, durva juice contains many vital nourishing factors and has come to be known as 'green blood'. It is cooling, astringent, demulcent, diuretic, ophthalmic, haemostatic and suppurative.

Profile

Botanical Name : Cynodon dactilon

Other Species : Panicum dactilon

Family : Gramineae (Poaceae)

Appearance : A perennial grass, used as fodder. Stem - slender, creeping, rooting at all nodes. Branches - erect. Leaves - narrowly linear. Fruit - oblong, laterally compressed grain.

Medicinal Parts : Roots, the whole plant.

Distribution : A very common weed throughout India and in tropical and warm temperate regions throughout the world. It is also one of the common grasses used on tennis lawns.

Ailments and Cure

Blood discharges from eyes - Boil ½ cup clean grass with an equal amount of the tender leaves of pomegranate in 2 cups of water till reduced to 1 cup. Strain and cool. Dose : ½ cup. Repeat after 2 hours.

Burning sensation in eyes – Boil 3 tbsp pulp of ash gourd along with 3 tbsp of cleaned grass in 2 cups of water till the volume is reduced to 1 cup. Dose ½ cup thrice daily.

Eye ailments, to strengthen eyesight – Extract the pure sap of cleaned grass and use as eye drops. (Caution : Take precautions to prevent infection.)

Eye ailments – Soak a handful of leaves in 1 teacup water. Add 1 tbsp milk. Drink with or without sugar.

10. Fenugreek

(Trigonella foenum-graecum)

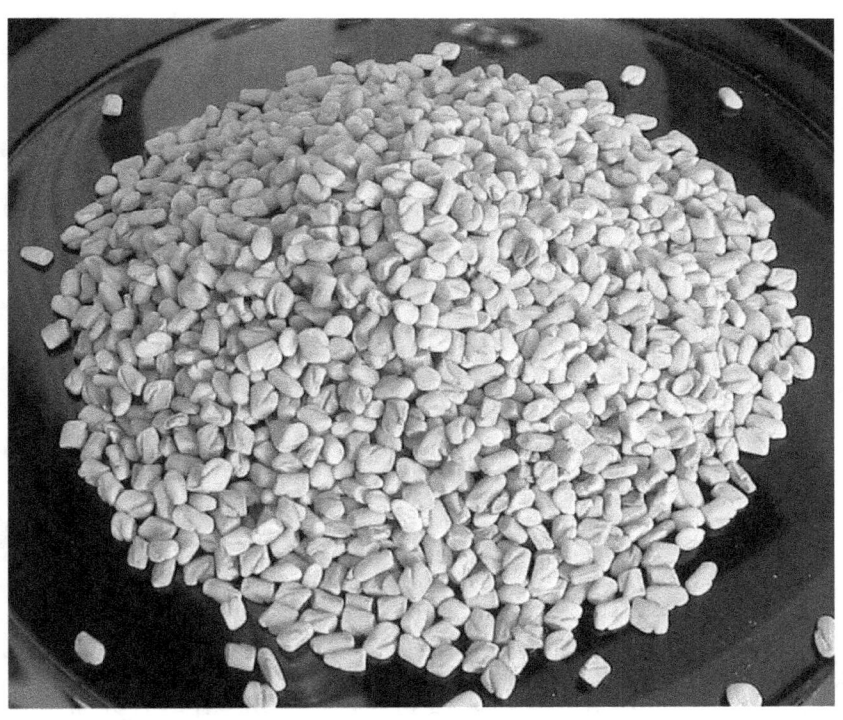

General

Fenugreek seeds are rich in iron and hence helpful in combating anaemia. It is also used to cure a number of common ailments – cough, fever, bronchitis, boils, ulcers..

Profile

Botanical Name : Trigonella foenum-graecum

Family : Leguminoseae

Appearance : Strong scented, erect, robust, annual herb with light green, pinnate, trifoliate leaves. Flowers – yellow. Pods – beaked. Seeds – brownish yellow with peculiar odour, oblong with deep groove across one corner.

Medicinal Parts : leaves, seeds

Distribution : Cultivated worldwide as a semi-arid crop.

Ailments and Cure

Burning sensation in eyes, failing eyesight - Mix equal quantities of fenugreek seed powder along-with shikakai powder for washing hair. Wash frequently.

Failing eyesight – Boil 1 cup leaves and eat with honey, twice daily.

11. <u>Fig</u>

(Ficus carica)

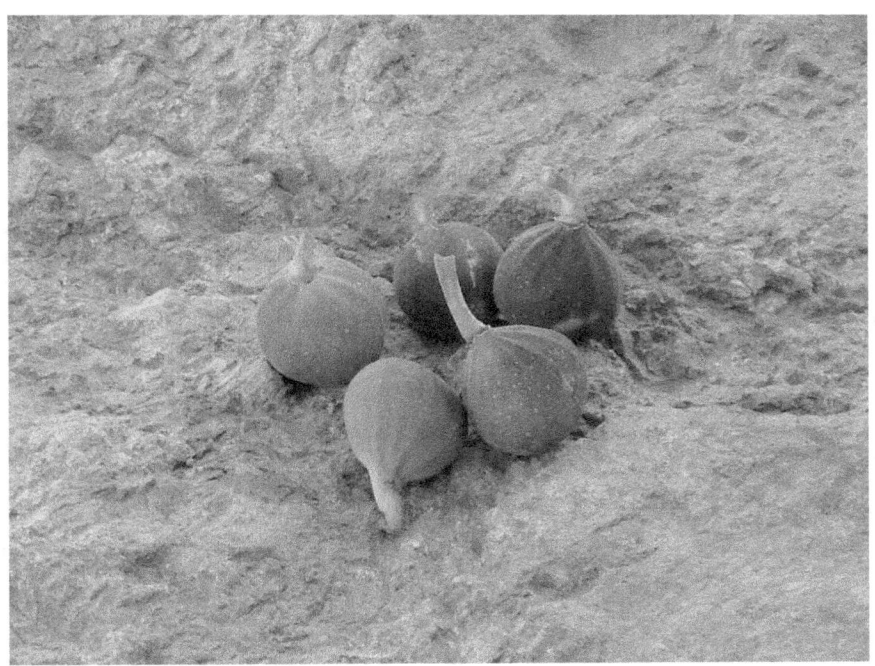

General

The fig tree which traces its origin to the Mediterranean region has enriched nutritional value. The dried fruits contain iron, copper and other minerals including trace elements like zinc, vitamin A and C, and a high concentration of invert sugar.

Profile

Botanical Name : Ficus carica

Family : Moraceae

Appearance : A small tree with alternate, long-petioled leaves. It bears its flowers inside a nearly closed receptacle. Fruits – pear shaped, fleshy. The stems and leaves contain an acrid milky juice.

Medicinal Parts : bark, leaves, leaf buds, roots, fruits (both fresh and dried), latex.

Distribution : Native to the Middle East and western Asia, it has been sought out and cultivated by man since ancient times, and is now widely grown throughout the temperate world.

Ailments and Cure

Eye problems due to acidity – Boil 2-3 figs with 1 tbsp raisins in 1 teacup milk. Drink every morning during breakfast.

12. Jamun

(Eugenia jambolana)

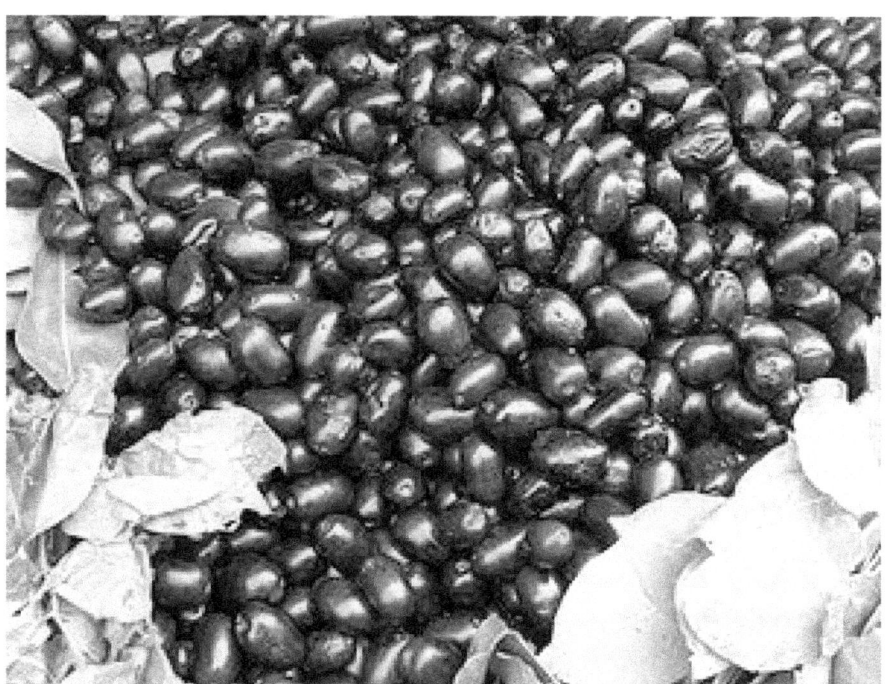

General

A fairly fast growing species, it can reach heights of up to 30 m and can live more than 100 years. Its dense foliage provides shade and is grown just for its ornamental value.

The wood is strong and is water resistant. Because of this it is used in railway sleepers and to install motors in wells. It is sometimes used to make cheap furniture and village dwellings though it is relatively hard to work on.

Profile

Botanical Name : Eugenia jambolana

Other species : Eugenia cumini, Syzygium cumini, Syzygium jambolanum

Family : Myrtaceae

Appearance : A large evergreen tree with light gray bark and dark gray patches. Leaves - smooth and oval in pairs. Flowers - small, numerous, sweet scented, dull white in bunches. Fruit - dark, purplish black, juicy when ripe. Seeds - round and smooth.

Medicinal Parts : Bark, fruit, kernel, leaves, seeds.

Distribution : Native to Bangladesh, India, Nepal, Pakistan, Sri Lanka, the Philippines, and Indonesia. The tree introduced in USA, Brazil, Suriname and Trinidad and Tobago.

Ailments and Cure

Burning sensation in eyes, watery eyes – Eat 5-10 jamun fruits after breakfast every day.

13. <u>Lime</u>

(Citrus aurantiifolia)

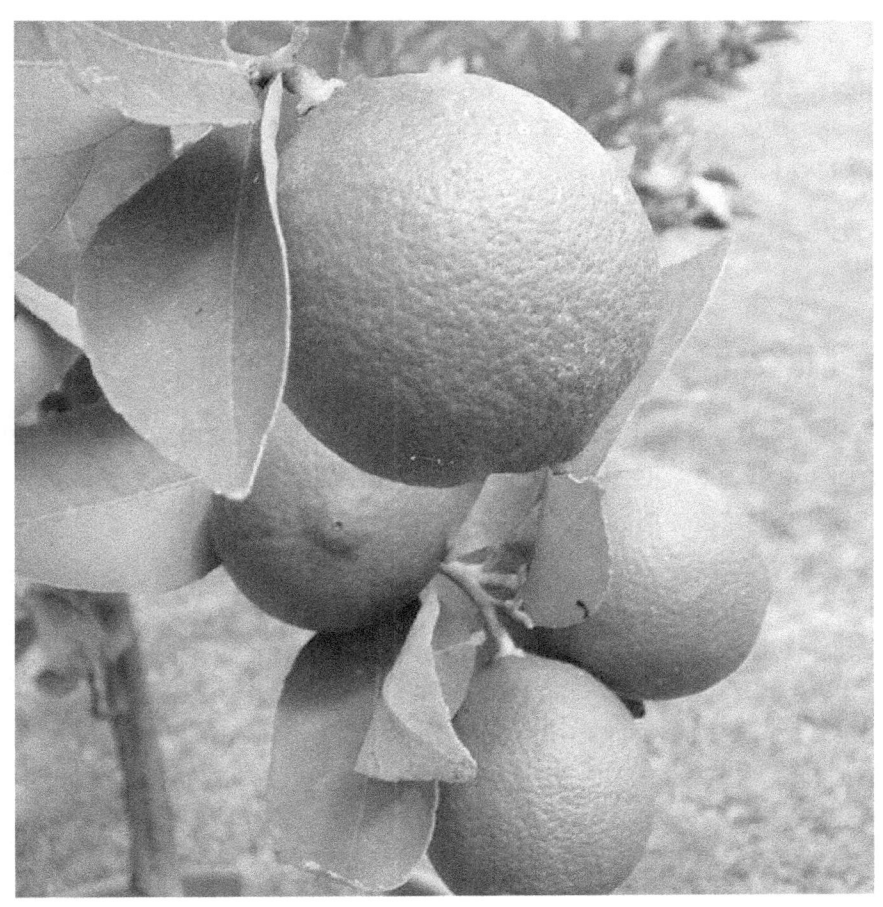

General

Lime is an easily available fruit, sour in taste and a rich source of vitamin C. They are grown all year round and are usually smaller and less sour than lemons.

Sour taste, in terms of herbalism, acts as a stimulant, promotes digestion, increases appetite and is a carminative (helps dispel flatus). It nourishes all tissues, except reproductive tissues.

Profile

Botanical Name : Citrus aurantiifolia, Limonia aurantiifolia

Family : Rutaceae

Appearance : A shrub or small tree. Fruit is typically round, green to yellow in colour, 3–6 cm in diameter, and containing sour and acidic pulp

Medicinal Parts : Fruits, Leaves, Roots

Distribution: Limes were first grown on a large scale in southern Iraq and Persia. Now, India tops the production list, followed by Mexico, Argentina, Brazil, and Spain.

Ailments and Cure

Eye diseases – One drop of lime juice put into the eyes every morning.

Watery eyes – Just touch the eyelids with a lime fruit softly several times.

14. Liquorice

(Glycyrrhiza glabra)

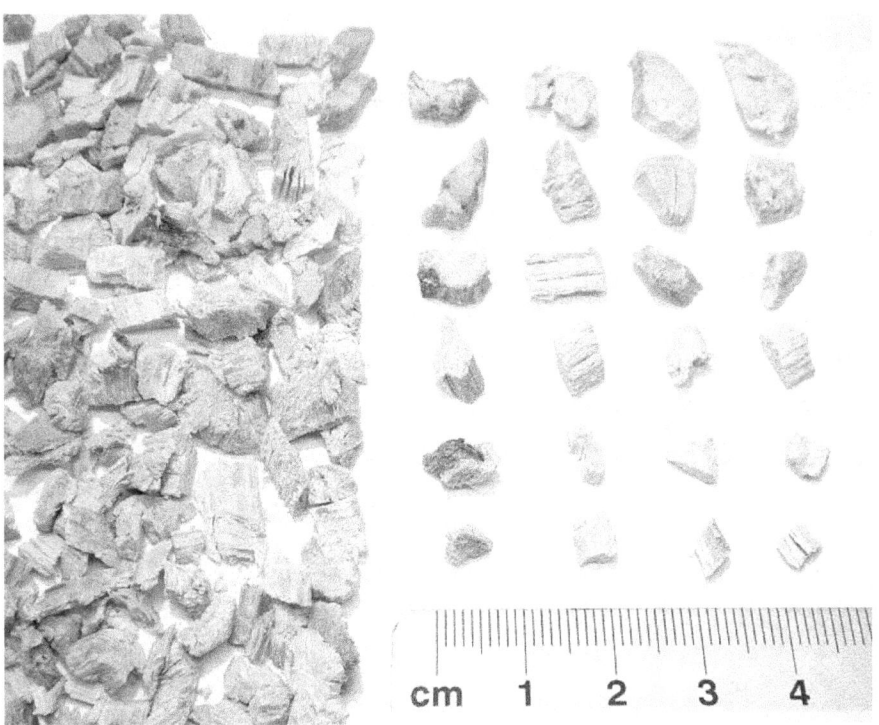

General

Liquorice or licorice is the root of Glycyrrhiza glabra from which a somewhat sweet flavor can be extracted.

It has been known for thousands of years for its medicinal value. It is used to strengthen muscles and bone, curing wounds, bronchial troubles, skin diseases, ulcer and jaundice.

Profile

Botanical Name : Glycyrrhiza glabra

Family : Fabaceae

Appearance : Perennial plant found wild. The woody rootstock is wrinkled and brown on the outside, yellow inside and tastes sweet. The stem which is round on the lower part and angular higher up bears alternate odd-pinnate leaves. Leaflets are ovate and dark green in color. Flowers – yellow or purple or violet. Pods – compressed.

Medicinal Parts : Rootstock(rhizome)

Distribution: Native to southern Europe and parts of Asia. Cultivated mostly in sub-Himalayan tracts.

Ailments and Cure

Aching eyes – Powder equal quantities of liquorice and cumin. Take ¼ tsp every day along with 1 tsp honey for a month.

To remove yellowness in the eyes – Very fine powder of liquorice is dusted into eyes. (Caution : Proper care is to be excercised.)

15. Onion

(Allium cepa)

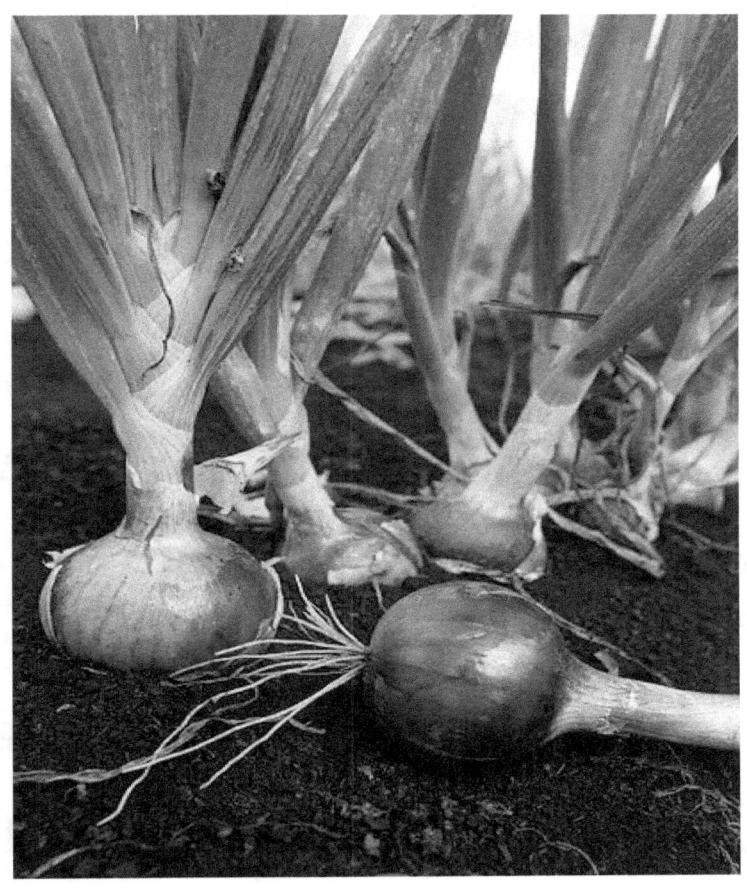

General

Onion is considered the oldest cultivated herb. Besides its bulbs, its green shoots, flowers and seeds – all are reputed to possess medicinal properties.

As an antiseptic, onion helps to end putrefactive and fermentative processes in the gastro-intestinal tracts.

Profile

Botanical Name : Allium cepa

Family : Liliaceae

Appearance : The plant consists of a prominent bulb, formed by thickening of the leaf base when mature. Leaves are long, linear and hollow. Florets are white.

Medicinal Parts : Bulb, shoots, flowers, seeds.

Distribution: Cultivated all over world. Major onion production comes from China, India, USA, Egypt, Iran, Turkey, Pakistan, Brazil, Russia and South Korea.

Ailments and Cure

Eyesight improvement – Use juice of onion flowers as eye drops.

And/or, Fry sliced onion shoots in butter/ghee and eat regularly.(Caution : This should not be given to children continuously).

16. Papaya

(Carica papaya)

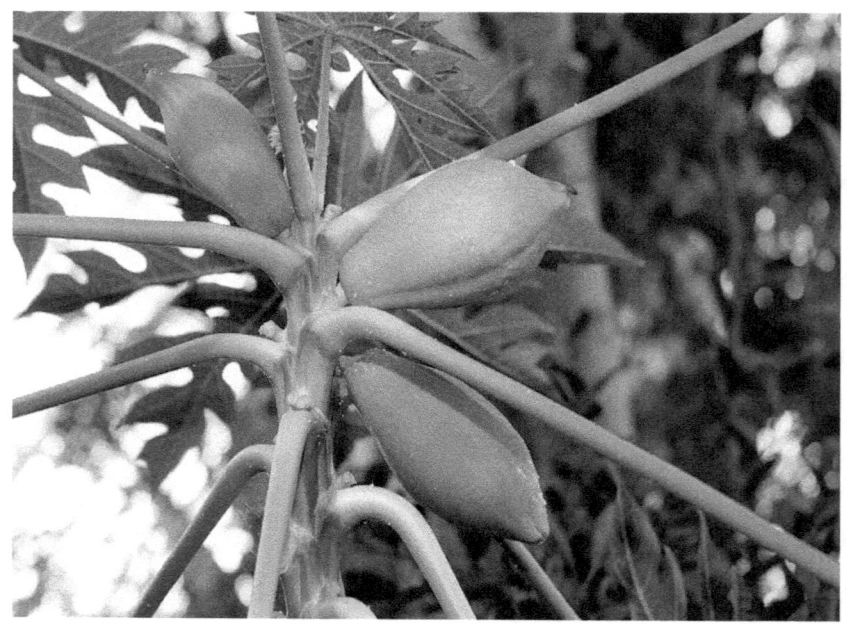

General

Nearly every inch of papaya tree possesses medicinal properties. Like the legendary apple, a papaya a day can also keep the doctor away.

Profile

Botanical Name : Carica papaya

Family : Caricaceae

Appearance : A tree having soft wood with palm like leaves. Male and female flowers are on separate trees. The fruit is large, oblong or nearly spherical fleshy berry with yellow orange rind like a gourd.

Medicinal Parts : Leaves, fruits(ripe or unripe), latex

Distribution : Originally from southern Mexico (particularly Chiapas and Veracruz), Central America, and northern South America, the papaya is now cultivated in most tropical countries.

Ailments and Cure

Eye diseases - Eat papayas frequently.

17. <u>Rose</u>

(Rosa centifolia)

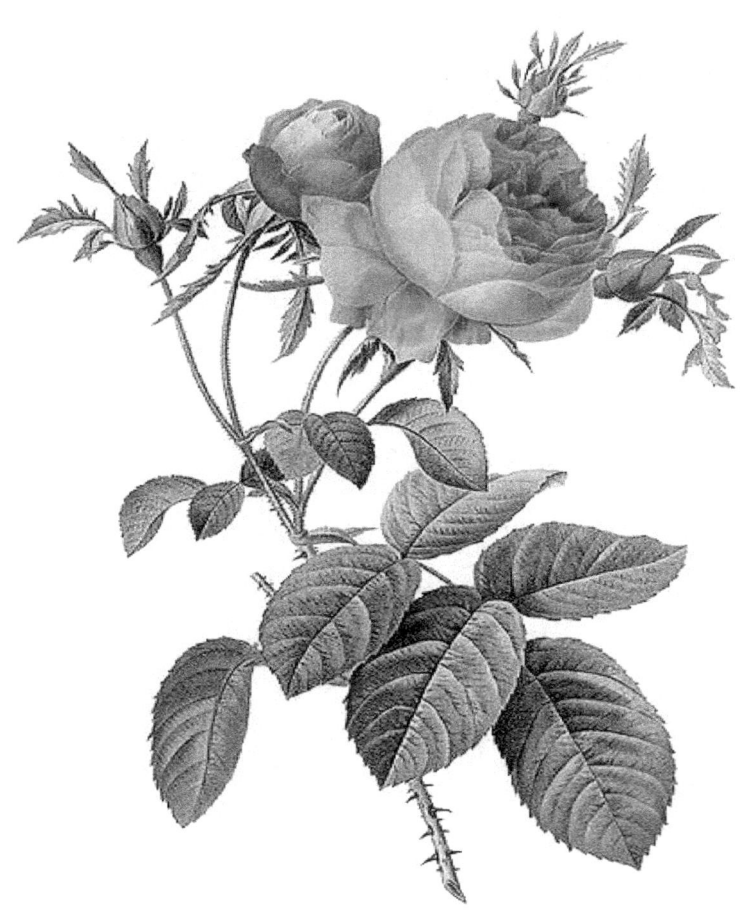

General

Rose cultivated in gardens for ornamental purposes are complex hybrids derived from many wild species. A few species are grown on a commercial scale which are used in perfumery and medicine.

Profile

Botanical Name : Rosa centifola

Appearance : A prickly shrub, white to crimson flowers. Stems bear alternate, odd-pinnate leaves. Flowers are usually single and five petaled in wild species, but often double in cultivated varieties.

Medicinal Parts : Flowers, rose-hips

Distribution : Most species are native to Asia, with smaller numbers native to Europe, North America, and northwest Africa.

Ailments and Cure

Burning sensation in eyes - Instil several drops of pure rose water in the affected eye.

And/or, Mix 1 tsp each rose water and onion juice. Drench clean cotton in this liquid and place on the closed eyes.

18. <u>Saunf (Fennel)</u>

(Foeniculum vulgare)

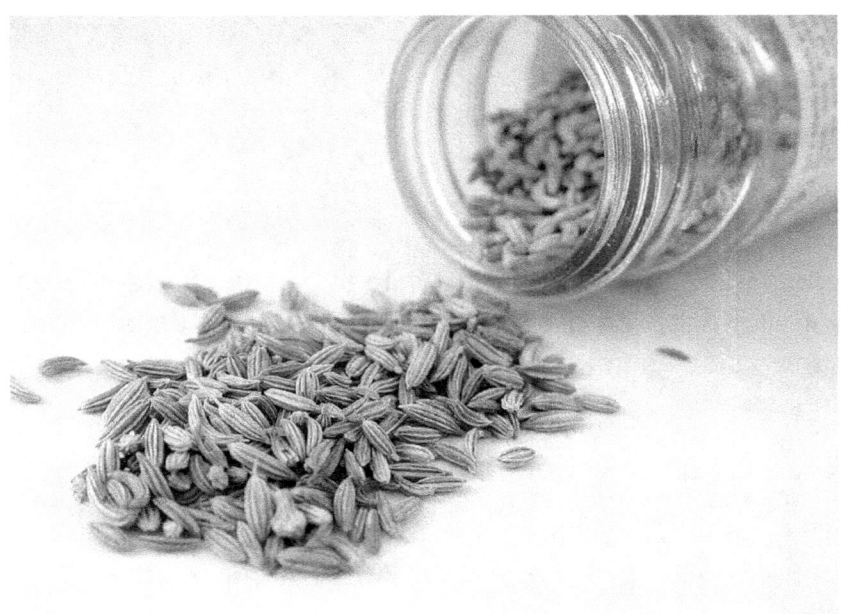

General

Saunf consists of the fruits of fennel, often wrongly called seeds. It constitutes an excellent remedy for a number of ailments.

Profile

Botanical Name : Foeniculum vulgare, Foeniculum officinale, Foeniculum capillaceum, Anethum foeniculum

Other Species : Fennel, Indian sweet fennel.

Family : Apiaceae (Formerly Umbelliferae)

Appearance : A tall glabrous aromatic herb. Leaves – pinnately decompound. Flowers – small, yellow, in umbels. Fruit – ellipsoid, 6-7 mm in length, greenish or yellowish brown.

Medicinal Parts : Roots, fruits(seeds)

Distribution : It is indigenous to the shores of the Mediterranean but has become widely naturalized in many parts of the world, especially on dry soils near the sea-coast and on riverbanks.

Ailments and Cure

Eye inflammation, strengthen eye muscles – Boil 2 tbsp saunf in 1 teacup water till it is reduced to half. Filter. Take 1 tbsp every morning and evening for a few days.

Use this filtrate to wash the eyes frequently to strengthen eye muscles and as a cleansing lotion for inflamed eyes.

Eye irritation, eye strain due to excessive reading or TV watching – Boil ½ tsp saunf in a cup of water till it is reduced to half. Cool. Use as eye drops (Caution : Beware of contamination).

19. <u>Sesame</u>

(Sesamum indicum)

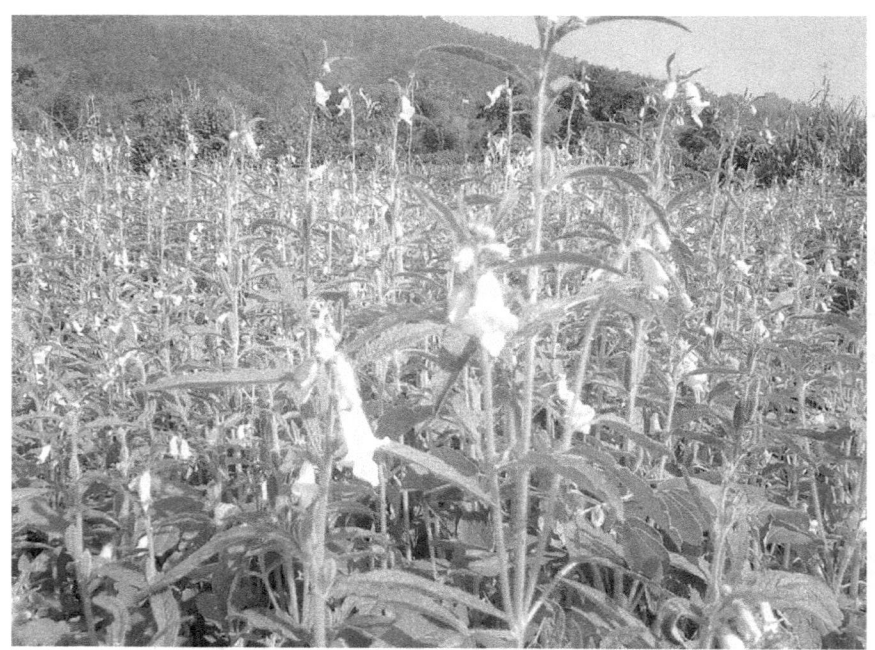

General

Sesame is a flowering plant and is cultivated for its edible seeds, which grow in pods.

Sesame seed is considered to be the oldest oilseed crop known, domesticated well over 5000 years ago. Sesame is very drought-tolerant. It has been called a survivor crop, with an ability to grow where most crops fail.

Profile

Botanical Name : Sesamum indicum

Family : Pedaliaceae

Appearance : Tall, erect, annual herb. Leaves ovate, grow alternately on the stem and are deeply veined. Flowers whitish yellow. Fruit is a two shelled pod which burst open when seeds are ripe. Seeds vary in color from yellowish white to black.

Medicinal Parts : Seeds, oil.

Distribution: It is widely naturalized in tropical regions around the world. Burma, India, and China account for 50 percent of global production.

Ailments and Cure

Burning sensation in the eyes – Mix the juice of bottle gourd and sesame oil (4:1) and heat till moisture is evaporated completely. Once cool, use it for massaging the head.

20. <u>Sweet Basil</u>

(Ocimum basilicum)

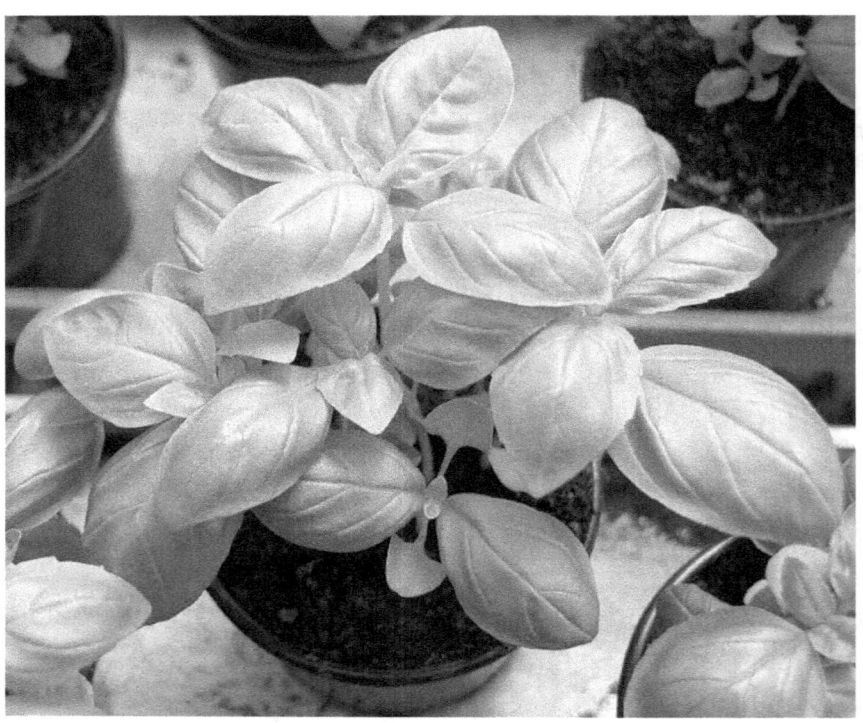

General

Basil, or Sweet Basil, originally from India, is a half-hardy annual plant, best known as a culinary herb.

Prominently featured in Italian cuisine, it also plays a major role in the Northeast Asian cuisine of Taiwan and the Southeast Asian cuisines of Indonesia, Thailand, Vietnam, Cambodia, and Laos.

Two most distinguishable characteristics of this family are the lip like corolla and the heavy smell of leaves. The characteristic odor of leaves is due to numerous dot like oil glands brimming with volatile oils. The aroma purifies the surroundings, making it the most sought after natural air fresheners that are easily grown in the garden.

Profile

Botanical Name : Ocimum basilicum

Family : Lamiaceae

Appearance : An aromatic herb with green or purplish branches. Leaves - simple, egg like, shiny. Flowers - 2-lipped, white or pale purple. Fruits - ellipsoid, black in color.

Medicinal Parts : Leaves, the whole plant.

Distribution : Basil is originally native to India and other tropical regions of Asia.

Ailments and Cure

Boil on eyelids (stye) – Rub a conch shell with the leaf juice of basil and pass gently over the stye.

21. Tamarind

(Tamarindus indica)

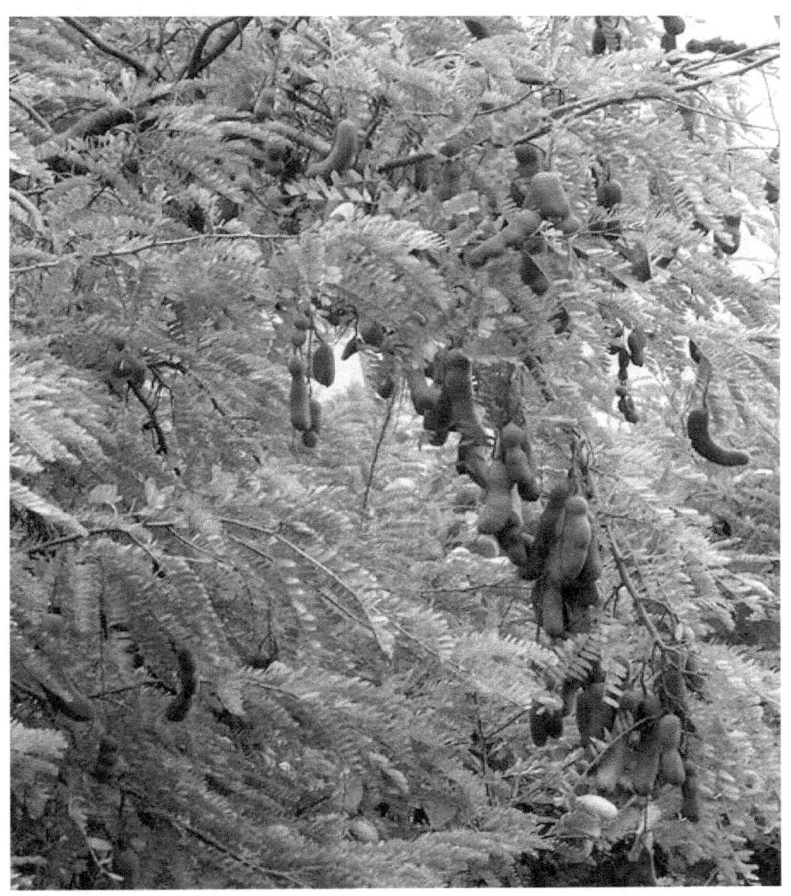

General

It is perhaps one of the most acidic naturally occurring substances, the principal acid being tartaric acid.

Tamarind is useful because of its anti-microbial and anti-bacterial properties. The tender leaves too fight worms. Apart from its use against germs, the fruit pulp also exhibits several medicinal properties - anthelmintic, carminative, digestive, laxative, and refrigerant.

Profile

Botanical Name : Tamarindus indica

Family : Leguminoseae

Appearance : A tree with small shiny leaflets. Flowers cream yellow to pinkish, in clusters. Pods - thick and oblong. Seeds - brown, compressed, embedded in a fibrous, fleshy, acid pulp.

Medicinal Parts : Bark, flowers, fruits, leaves, seeds, kernel.

Distribution: Native to tropical Africa, the tree is quite common in India.

Ailments and Cure

Eye diseases – Grind a handful of clean flowers into a fine paste and apply around the eyes at bedtime.

Painful eyes, redness in the eyes – Grind a handful of flowers into a fine paste and apply over the eyes before going to bed.

Swelling in the eyes – Use a poultice of flowers.

22. <u>Turmeric</u>

(Curcuma longa)

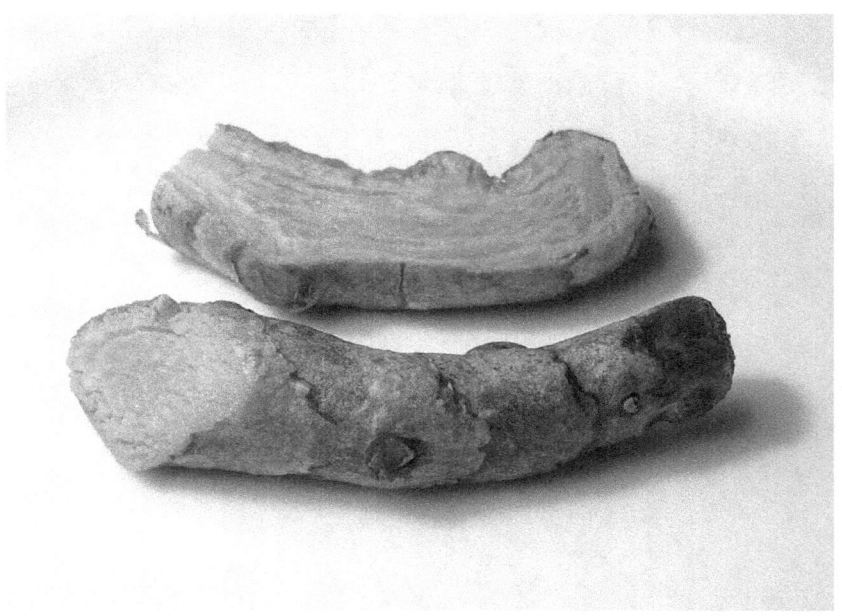

General

The turmeric which is available commercially for cooking purposes is the boiled, debarked rootstock which has lost many of its miraculous medicinal properties. The raw, dried rootstock of the plant should therefore be preferred.

Profile

Botanical Name : Curcuma longa, Curcuma domestica

Family : Zingiberaceae

Appearance : The spice turmeric consists of dried, boiled, cleaned, and polished rootstock of the plant. The plant has a large tuft of leaves and spikes with pale green flowering bracts, covering yellow flowers.

Medicinal Parts : Rootstock (rhizome)

Distribution : India and Pakistan are significant producers of turmeric.

Ailments and Cure

Eye diseases – Boil 1 tsp turmeric powder thoroughly in 2 teacups water till it is reduced to half. Allow to cool. A few drops of this cold infusion is used as eye drops.

Ophthalmia – Extract juice from turmeric rhizomes and use as eye drops.

23. Vasaka

(Adhatoda vasica)

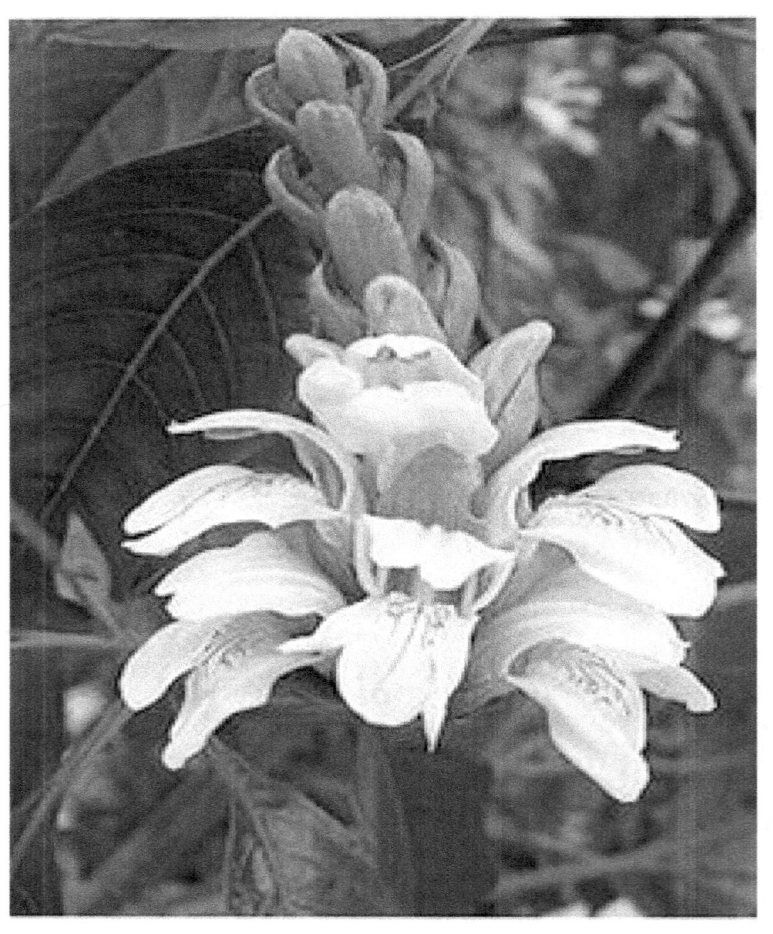

General

Vasaka grows in abundance in the lower reaches of the Himalayas. Sometimes it is cultivated as a hedge plant. The drug vasaka comes from fresh or dried leaves of the plant, and is administered in form of juice, syrup or decoction.

Profile

Botanical Name : Adhatoda vasica

Other Species : Adhatoda zeylanica, Justicia adhatoda

Family : Acanthaceae

Appearance : Tall, dense, ever green shrub. Leaves - large, lance shaped, somewhat resembling mango leaves. Fruit - a capsule with 4 seeds. Flowers - white or purple.

Medicinal Parts : Flowers, leaves, roots, and bark

Distribution : The plant grows wild in abundance all over Sri Lanka, Nepal, India, and the Pothohar region of Pakistan, particularly in the Pharwala area.

Ailments and Cure

Eye diseases – Fry some flowers in a little ghee/butter. Allow to cool. Apply on closed eyes and wrap with a napkin. Allow it to remain for 15-20 minutes.

24. Vibhitaki

(Terminalia bellirica)

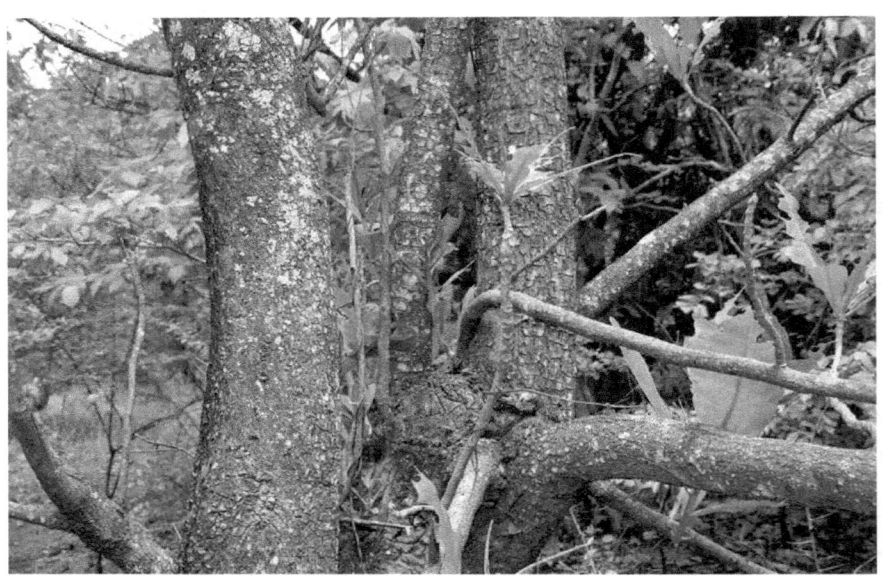

General

The fruits of vibhitaki exhibit hypotensive, purgative and choleretic activities. Its kernel is edible and is considered to have narcotic and aphrodisiac effects. It is prescribed in a variety of diseases : anaemia, cough, fever, asthma, diarrhoea, dysentery, biliousness, diseases of eyes, nose and throat etc. It stimulates hair growth, cures leprosy, and purifies the blood.

Profile

Botanical Name : Terminalia bellirica

Family : Combretaceae

Appearance : A long avene tree with ash-grey bark, with patches of blue. Leaves - elliptic, crowded towards the ends of branches. Flowers - pale, greenish yellow with an offensive odour. Fruit - grey to light violet when fresh, turning light brown later.

Medicinal Parts : Bark, fruits, leaves.

Distribution: Vibhitaki is a large deciduous tree common on plains and lower hills in Southeast Asia, where it is also grown as an avenue tree.

Ailments and Cure

To impart brightness in eyes – Roast the rind and powder. Take 1/2 tsp with 1 tsp each honey and white sugar for three months.

Some Important Guidelines

1. Preparation

When the herb is extremely bitter, sour, astringent or in powdered form, it can be mixed with honey, jaggery, sugar, candy etc.

2. Dosage

The quantity of dose can vary from one person to another based on individual age, physical build, and reaction of patient to a particular formulation.

The dosage prescribed in this book is meant for fully grown and mature patients. The dose should be increased/decreased for each patient keeping in mind individual patient's constitution.

3. Effectiveness

The contents of a herbal plant part varies widely due to factors such as climate, altitude, latitude, soil type, nutrition, temperature, relative humidity, time of plucking, packaging, storage etc. Hence the effectiveness of herb for treating an ailment may vary in different cases.

Patient needs to keep in mind this inherent weakness of herbal effectiveness, and be prepared to continue the treatment for a little longer time.

Other Books That May Interest You

Herbs That Cure:

Anaemia
Asthma
Bad Breath
Bronchitis
Constipation
Diabetes
Diarrhoea
ENT Problems
Fatigue
Flatulence
Genito-Urinal disorders
Haemorrhoids
Hair Loss
Heart Problems
Insomnia
Joints Pain
Leucoderma
Obesity
Pimples
Psoriasis
Rheumatism
Sexual Debility
Skin Diseases
Stomach Disorders
Toothache
Venereal Diseases
Wrinkles

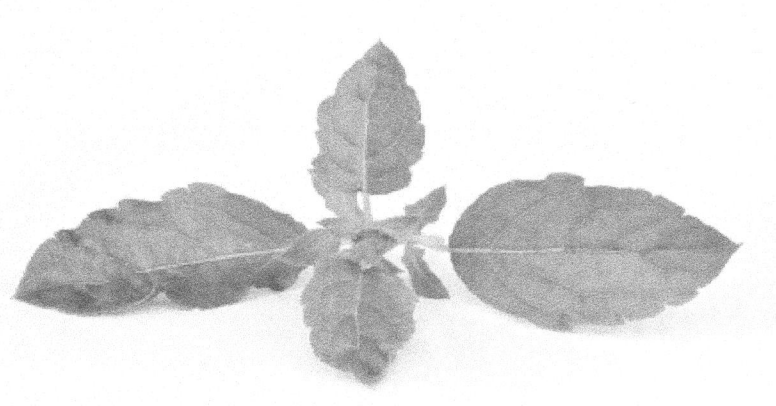

www.ingramcontent.com/pod-product-compliance
Lightning Source LLC
Chambersburg PA
CBHW070614290526
45790CB00002B/904